TYPE 2 DAIBETES COOKBOOK SENIORS

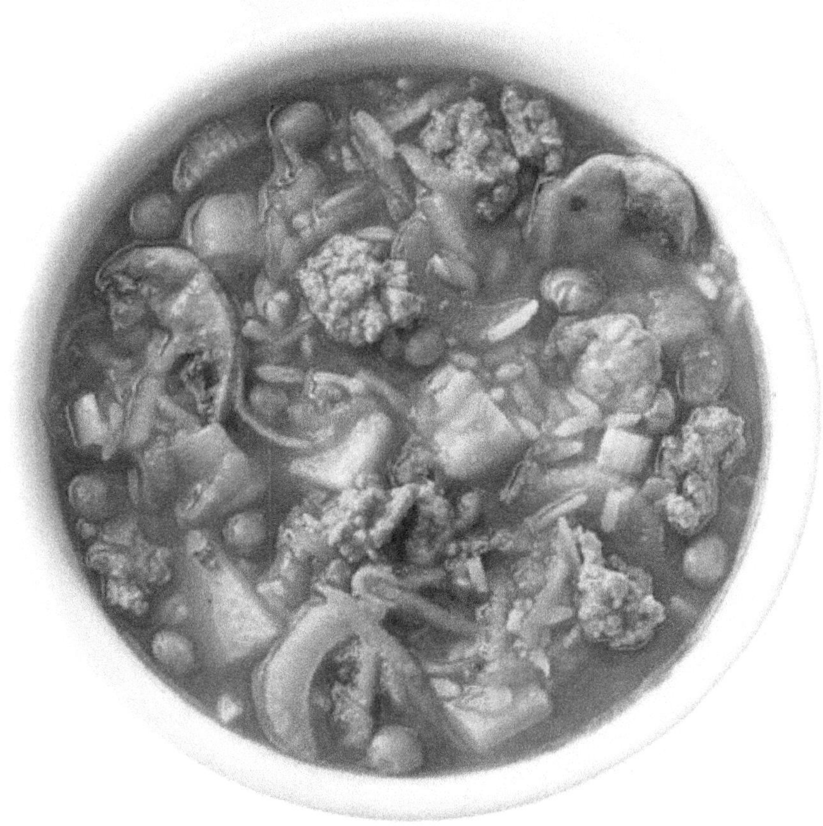

LORENE PEACHEY

TABLE OF CONTENTS

OTHER BOOKS BY THE AUTHOR

MEDITERRANEAN AIR FRYER COOKBOOK FOR BEGINNERS

LOW SODIUM SLOW COOKER COOKBOOK

MEDITERRANEAN DIET COOKBOOK FOR NEWBIES 2024

DIABETIC RENAL DIET COOKBOOK FOR NEWLY DAIGNOSED

RENAL DIET AIR FRYER COOKBOOK FOR SENIORS

KIDNEY DISEASE DIET COOKBOOK FOR WOMEN

INTRODUCTION

In the quiet town of Harmony Ville, where the sun sets over amber fields and folks share stories on the porch swing, I, Nutritionist Lorene Peachey, stumbled upon a culinary journey that would transform lives. Let me share with you the heartwarming tale of Martha Thompson, a sweet soul from our community who, like many, found herself trapped in the clutches of type 2 diabetes.

Martha, a lively woman with a contagious laugh and a heart as big as the Mississippi, had tried every cookbook on the market. From the famous to the forgotten, she embraced them all, with each turn of the page carrying the hope of discovering a recipe that could dance with her taste buds and mend her health. But, alas, the results were far from the culinary symphony she yearned for.

One day, as the sun dipped below the horizon, casting shadows on her quaint kitchen, Martha stumbled upon my cookbook, "Type 2 Diabetes Cookbook for Seniors." Intrigued, she decided to embark on a flavourful journey, fuelled not only by the desire for delicious meals but also the hope for a healthier, more vibrant life.

The pages of my cookbook, much like the fields of Harmony Ville in spring, burst forth with colours, aromas, and stories of transformation. Martha dove in, her apron a canvas for culinary creations waiting to unfold. From the first sizzle of the pan to the aroma that filled her kitchen, Martha's heart danced to a new rhythm — one of balance, vitality, and fulfillment.

As Martha dived into my recipes, something magical began to happen. Her blood sugar levels, once as unpredictable as a summer storm, steadied into a gentle breeze. The weight that had lingered on her shoulders like a heavy secret started to lift, and the sparkle returned to her eyes. With each dish, she discovered a symphony of Flavors that whispered tales of nourishment and restoration.

Oh, how she delighted in the Quinoa Salad with Lemon Herb Vinaigrette, a melody of textures and Flavors that made her taste buds twirl. And who could forget the Grilled Lemon Garlic Chicken with Roasted Vegetables, a savory sonnet that sang of health and satisfaction? Martha found herself embracing breakfasts of Berry Citrus Smoothie Bowls that burst with the sweetness of dawn, bringing a new sunrise to her health.

But the true crescendo in Martha's journey was the discovery of more than just recipes. The benefits of embracing healthy diabetes foods were not confined to her plate; they seeped into every facet of her life. Suddenly, her steps were lighter, her laughter contagious, and her energy infectious. The transformation was not merely physical but a soulful metamorphosis that touched the very core of her being.

In the midst of her rediscovery, Martha began to ponder the questions that my cookbook gently nudged her towards. What does it mean to Savor life to the fullest? How does the food we choose define the melody of our existence? And most importantly, why do we wait until our health calls for a symphony of renewal before we start dancing to its rhythm?

Martha's journey, however, was not just a tale of success; it was a stark reminder of the dangers that lurk in the shadows of unhealthy choices. The consequences of indulging in a diet laden with processed sugars and unhealthy fats echoed like a haunting refrain in her memories. The dangers of diabetes, the silent predator that creeps into the lives of many, were not lost on her.

As Martha's story unfolded, so did the advantages and benefits of having my cookbook in her hands. The recipes were not just a collection of ingredients; they were a lifeline. They offered not only culinary delight but a roadmap to a healthier, more vibrant future. The friendly tone of the cookbook became a comforting companion, guiding Martha through the labyrinth of nutritious choices.

And so, dear reader, as you embark on this journey with me through " Type 2 Diabetes Cookbook for Seniors," know that you hold more than just a cookbook. You hold the key to a symphony of Flavors that can rejuvenate not just your body but your entire way of life. Ask yourself: What would it mean to Savor every bite, to dance with the rhythm of wholesome living? How could a cookbook become a companion in your journey to renewed health and joy?

As you leaf through the pages, imagine the aroma that wafts from each recipe, the vibrant colours that fill your plate, and the stories of transformation that echo in every bite. Let this cookbook be your guide, your muse, and your friend. For in each recipe lies not just the promise of a delicious meal but the invitation to embrace a life filled with vitality, balance, and the sweet melody of renewal.

Contact the Author

Thank you for reading my book! I would love to hear from you, whether you have feedback, questions, or just want to share your thoughts. Your feedback means a lot to me and helps me improve as a writer.

Please don't hesitate to reach out to me through

lorenepeachey@gmail.com

I look forward to connecting with my readers and appreciate your support in this literary journey. Your thoughts and comments are valuable to me.

CHAPTER 1

UNDERSTANDING TYPE 2 DIABETES

Type 2 diabetes is a chronic condition that affects how your body utilizes insulin, a hormone that regulates blood sugar. In individuals with type 2 diabetes, the body either doesn't produce enough insulin or becomes resistant to its effects. This leads to elevated blood sugar levels, which, if left uncontrolled, can result in various health complications.

Managing type 2 diabetes involves making lifestyle changes, including adopting a healthy diet, regular physical activity, and, in some cases, medication. Regular monitoring of blood sugar levels is crucial to ensuring effective management and preventing complications.

Importance of a Diabetes-Friendly Diet:

A diabetes-friendly diet is essential for individuals with type 2 diabetes to help regulate blood sugar levels and maintain overall health. Here are key components of a diabetes-friendly diet:

Carbohydrate Control: Monitor and regulate carbohydrate intake, focusing on complex carbohydrates with a low glycemic index. This helps in avoiding rapid spikes in blood sugar levels.

Portion Control: Controlling portion sizes is vital to managing calorie intake and blood sugar levels. Eating smaller, balanced meals throughout the day can help stabilize energy levels.

Healthy Fats: Choose sources of healthy fats, such as avocados, nuts, and olive oil, while limiting saturated and trans fats. This supports heart health, a common concern for individuals with diabetes.

Lean Proteins: Include lean protein sources like poultry, fish, beans, and tofu in your diet. Protein helps maintain muscle mass and provides a feeling of fullness.

Fiber-Rich Foods: Opt for high-fiber foods like whole grains, fruits, vegetables, and legumes. Fiber aids in digestion, helps control blood sugar levels, and promotes a feeling of satiety.

Tips for Seniors Managing Diabetes:

Seniors with diabetes face unique challenges in managing their condition. Here are some tips to help them effectively manage type 2 diabetes:

Regular Monitoring: Stay vigilant with blood sugar monitoring. Regular checks help identify trends and allow for timely adjustments to medication or lifestyle.

Medication Adherence: Take medications as prescribed by healthcare professionals. Set up a routine and use pill organizers to help remember doses.

Balanced Meals: Plan well-balanced meals that incorporate a variety of nutrient-rich foods. Consider consulting a dietitian for personalized meal planning.

Stay Active: Engage in regular physical activity appropriate for your fitness level. Activities like walking, swimming, or chair exercises can be beneficial.

Regular Health Checkups: Schedule regular checkups with healthcare providers to monitor overall health, including eye exams, blood pressure checks, and cholesterol levels.

Hydration: Stay adequately hydrated. Water is a healthy beverage choice that helps regulate blood sugar levels and supports overall well-being.

By understanding type 2 diabetes, embracing a diabetes-friendly diet, and implementing practical tips, seniors can effectively manage their condition and lead a healthier, more active life.

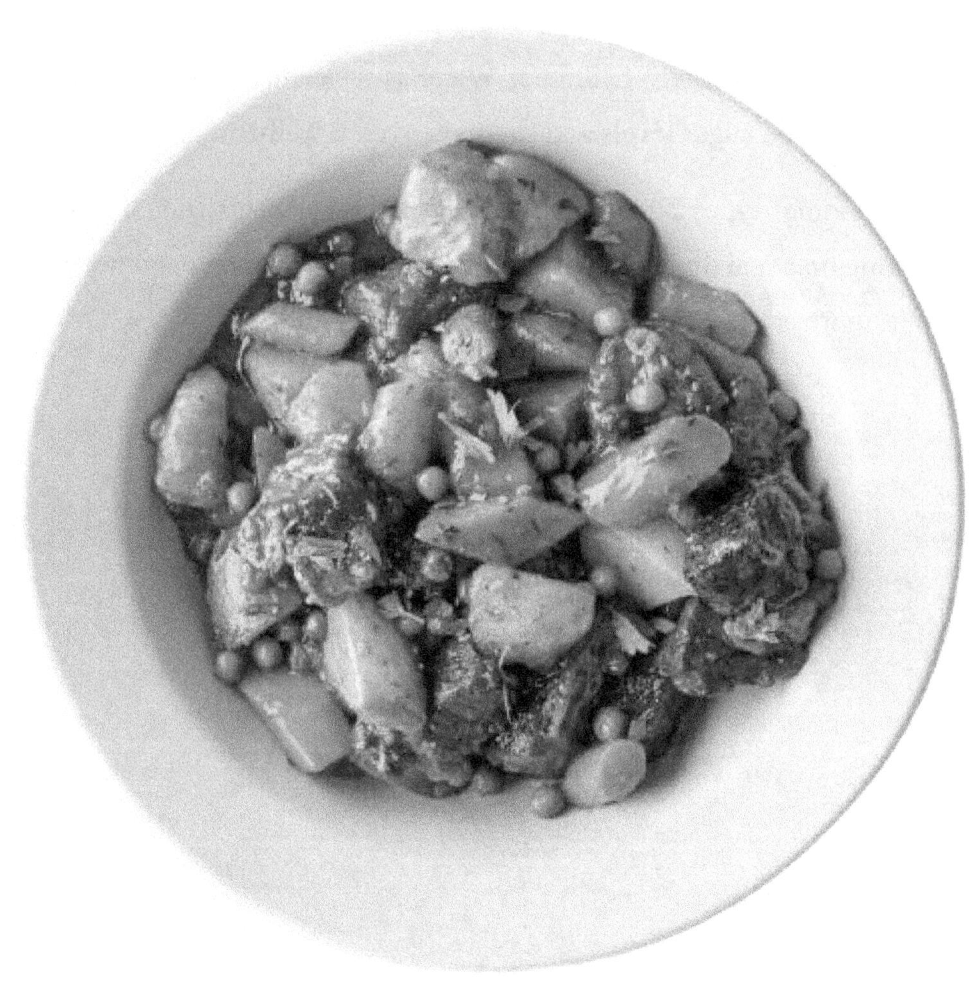

CHAPTER 1

BREAKFAST DELIGHTS

Oat-Free Chia Pudding with Berries and Almonds

Cooking Time: 5 minutes

Serving: 1

Ingredients:

- ✓ 2 tablespoons chia seeds
- ✓ 1/2 cup unsweetened almond milk
- ✓ 1/4 cup mixed berries
- ✓ 1 tablespoon sliced almonds.
- ✓ 1 teaspoon sugar-free sweetener

Instructions:

1. Mix chia seeds and almond milk; refrigerate for 4 hours or overnight.
2. Top with berries, almonds, and sweetener before serving.

Nutritional Information:

250 calories, 15g carbs, 8g protein, 15g fat, 8g fiber.

Chia seeds provide fiber and healthy fats for a filling breakfast.

Low-Carb Greek Yogurt Parfait

Cooking Time: 5 minutes

Serving: 1

Ingredients:

- ✓ 1/2 cup plain Greek yogurt.
- ✓ 1/4 cup blueberries
- ✓ 1 tablespoon chopped walnuts.
- ✓ 1 teaspoon flaxseeds
- ✓ 1 teaspoon sugar-free vanilla extract

Instructions:

1. Layer yogurt with blueberries, walnuts, and flaxseeds.
2. Drizzle with vanilla extract.

Nutritional Information:

200 calories, 10g carbs, 15g protein, 12g fat, 5g fiber.

Greek yogurt provides protein, while flaxseeds offer omega-3 fatty acids.

Avocado and Smoked Salmon Wrap

Cooking Time: 8 minutes

Serving: 1

Ingredients:

- ✓ 1 low-carb whole-grain wrap
- ✓ 1/2 ripe avocado, sliced.
- ✓ 2 ounces smoked salmon.
- ✓ 1 tablespoon cream cheese
- ✓ 1 teaspoon capers

Instructions:

1. Spread cream cheese on the wrap; add avocado, salmon, and capers.
2. Roll up and slice before serving.

Nutritional Information:

280 calories, 15g carbs, 20g protein, 18g fat, 8g fiber.

Healthy fats from avocado and omega-3s from salmon support heart health.

Spinach and Feta Omelets

Cooking Time: 10 minutes

Serving: 1

Ingredients:

- ✓ 2 large eggs, beaten.
- ✓ 1/2 cup fresh spinach, chopped.
- ✓ 2 tablespoons feta cheese, crumbled.
- ✓ 1/4 cup cherry tomatoes, halved.
- ✓ 1 teaspoon olive oil

Instructions:

1. Sauté spinach and tomatoes in olive oil until wilted.
2. Pour beaten eggs over vegetables, sprinkle with feta, and cook until set.

Nutritional Information:

220 calories, 5g carbs, 18g protein, 14g fat, 2g fiber.

High protein and low carb, perfect for stabilizing blood sugar.

Almond Flour Pancakes

Cooking Time: 15 minutes

Serving: 2

Ingredients:

- ✓ 1 cup almond flour
- ✓ 2 eggs
- ✓ 1/2 cup unsweetened almond milk
- ✓ 1 teaspoon baking powder
- ✓ 1 tablespoon melted butter.

Instructions:

1. Mix almond flour, eggs, almond milk, and baking powder.
2. Cook small pancakes in butter until golden brown.

Nutritional Information:

180 calories, 6g carbs, 9g protein, 15g fat, 3g fiber.

Low-carb alternative to traditional pancakes, rich in almond's healthy fats.

Vegetable and Cheese Frittata

Cooking Time: 12 minutes

Serving: 1

Ingredients:

- ✓ 2 large eggs, beaten.
- ✓ 1/4 cup bell peppers, diced.
- ✓ 1/4 cup zucchini, sliced.
- ✓ 2 tablespoons shredded cheddar cheese
- ✓ 1 teaspoon olive oil

Instructions:

1. Sauté bell peppers and zucchini in olive oil until softened.
2. Pour beaten eggs over vegetables, add cheese, and cook until set.

Nutritional Information:

240 calories, 7g carbs, 15g protein, 17g fat, 2g fiber.

Packed with veggies, this frittata is a nutrient-dense, low-carb breakfast.

Cauliflower Hash Browns

Cooking Time: 15 minutes

Serving: 2

Ingredients:

- ✓ 2 cups grated cauliflower.
- ✓ 1 egg
- ✓ 2 tablespoons almond flour
- ✓ 1/2 teaspoon garlic powder
- ✓ Salt and pepper to taste

Instructions:

1. Mix cauliflower, egg, almond flour, garlic powder, salt, and pepper.
2. Form into patties and cook until golden brown.

Nutritional Information:

160 calories, 8g carbs, 9g protein, 11g fat, 3g fiber.

A low-carb alternative to traditional hash browns, using nutrient-rich cauliflower.

Berry Protein Smoothie Bowl

Preparation Time: 10 minutes

Serving: 1

Ingredients:

- ✓ 1/2 cup frozen berries
- ✓ 1 scoop vanilla protein powder
- ✓ 1/2 cup unsweetened almond milk
- ✓ 1 tablespoon chia seeds
- ✓ 1 tablespoon unsweetened coconut flakes

Instructions:

1. Blend berries, protein powder, and almond milk until smooth.
2. Pour into a bowl, top with chia seeds and coconut flakes.

Nutritional Information:

220 calories, 12g carbs, 20g protein, 10g fat, 6g fiber.

A protein-packed, low-carb smoothie bowl with the goodness of berries.

Turkey and Veggie Breakfast Skillet

Cooking Time: 15 minutes

Serving: 1

Ingredients:

- ✓ 3 oz ground turkey
- ✓ 1/4 cup broccoli, chopped.
- ✓ 1/4 cup red bell pepper, diced.
- ✓ 1/4 cup onion, chopped.
- ✓ 1 tablespoon olive oil

Instructions:

1. Cook turkey in olive oil until browned.
2. Add veggies and sauté until tender.

Nutritional Information:

280 calories, 8g carbs, 22g protein, 18g fat, 3g fiber.

A savory, high-protein skillet to kickstart your day.

Coconut Flour Pancakes

Cooking Time: 12 minutes

Serving: 2

Ingredients:

- ✓ 1/2 cup coconut flour
- ✓ 2 eggs
- ✓ 1/2 cup unsweetened coconut milk
- ✓ 1/2 teaspoon baking powder
- ✓ 1 tablespoon coconut oil (for cooking)

Instructions:

1. Mix coconut flour, eggs, coconut milk, and baking powder.
2. Cook small pancakes in coconut oil until golden brown.

Nutritional Information:

200 calories, 10g carbs, 8g protein, 14g fat, 5g fiber.

A coconut-flavored, low-carb alternative for pancake lovers.

Mushroom and Spinach Egg Muffins

Cooking Time: 20 minutes

Serving: 2

Ingredients:

- ✓ 4 large eggs, beaten.
- ✓ 1/2 cup mushrooms, diced.
- ✓ 1/2 cup spinach, chopped.
- ✓ 1/4 cup feta cheese, crumbled.
- ✓ Salt and pepper to taste

Instructions:

1. Mix eggs, mushrooms, spinach, feta, salt, and pepper.
2. Pour into muffin cups and bake until set.

Nutritional Information:

180 calories, 6g carbs, 12g protein, 11g fat, 2g fiber.

Convenient egg muffins with the earthy flavors of mushrooms and spinach.

Zucchini and Bacon Breakfast Casserole

Cooking Time: 25 minutes

Serving: 4

Ingredients:

- ✓ 4 cups zucchini, grated.
- ✓ 6 slices bacon cooked and crumbled.
- ✓ 1/2 cup cheddar cheese, shredded.
- ✓ 1/4 cup green onions, chopped.
- ✓ 4 eggs, beaten.

Instructions:

1. Combine zucchini, bacon, cheese, and green onions in a baking dish.
2. Pour beaten eggs over the mixture and bake until set.

Nutritional Information:

280 calories, 8g carbs, 18g protein, 20g fat, 3g fiber.

A flavorful casserole with the goodness of zucchini and bacon.

Low-Carb Breakfast Burrito Bowl

Cooking Time: 15 minutes

Serving: 1

Ingredients:

- ✓ 2 scrambled eggs
- ✓ 1/4 cup black beans drained and rinsed.
- ✓ 1/4 cup diced tomatoes.
- ✓ 1/4 cup avocado, sliced.
- ✓ 1 tablespoon salsa

Instructions:

1. Assemble eggs, black beans, tomatoes, and avocado in a bowl.
2. Top with salsa before serving.

Nutritional Information:

260 calories, 12g carbs, 18g protein, 15g fat, 6g fiber.

A satisfying burrito bowl without the carb-heavy tortilla.

Cottage Cheese and Walnut Stuffed Peppers

Preparation Time: 10 minutes

Serving: 2

Ingredients:

- ✓ 1 cup cottage cheese
- ✓ 1/4 cup walnuts, chopped.
- ✓ 1/4 teaspoon cinnamon
- ✓ 1/4 teaspoon vanilla extract
- ✓ 2 bell peppers, halved.

Instructions:

1. Mix cottage cheese, walnuts, cinnamon, and vanilla extract.
2. Stuff bell peppers with the mixture.

Nutritional Information:

220 calories, 10g carbs, 15g protein, 12g fat, 3g fiber.

A unique, protein-packed breakfast with a touch of sweetness.

Salmon and Cream Cheese Cucumber Rolls

Preparation Time: 10 minutes

Serving: 2

Ingredients:

- ✓ 4 ounces smoked salmon.
- ✓ 1/4 cup cream cheese
- ✓ 1 cucumber sliced lengthwise.
- ✓ Fresh dill for garnish

Instructions:

1. Spread cream cheese on cucumber slices.
2. Roll smoked salmon around the cucumber slices and garnish with fresh dill.

Nutritional Information:

240 calories, 5g carbs, 18g protein, 16g fat, 2g fiber.

A refreshing, low-carb alternative to traditional bagel and lox.

Chia Seed and Berry Smoothie

Preparation Time: 8 minutes

Serving: 1

Ingredients:

- ✓ 1 cup unsweetened almond milk
- ✓ 2 tablespoons chia seeds
- ✓ 1/2 cup mixed berries
- ✓ 1 scoop vanilla protein powder
- ✓ Ice cubes (optional)

Instructions:

1. Blend almond milk, chia seeds, berries, and protein powder until smooth.
2. Add ice cubes if desired and blend again.

Nutritional Information:

220 calories, 10g carbs, 20g protein, 10g fat, 8g fiber.

A protein-packed smoothie with chia seeds for added texture and fiber.

Egg and Veggie Breakfast Wrap

Cooking Time: 10 minutes

Serving: 1

Ingredients:

- ✓ 2 large eggs, scrambled.
- ✓ 1/4 cup bell peppers, sliced.
- ✓ 1/4 cup spinach leaves
- ✓ 1 low-carb whole-grain wrap
- ✓ 1 tablespoon feta cheese, crumbled.

Instructions:

1. Cook scrambled eggs, bell peppers, and spinach in a pan.
2. Fill the wrap with the cooked mixture, top with feta, and fold.

Nutritional Information:

250 calories, 12g carbs, 18g protein, 14g fat, 5g fiber.

A quick and satisfying breakfast wrap loaded with veggies.

Cauliflower and Broccoli Breakfast Bowl

Cooking Time: 12 minutes

Serving: 1

Ingredients:

- ✓ 1 cup cauliflower rice
- ✓ 1/2 cup broccoli florets
- ✓ 1 tablespoon olive oil
- ✓ 2 eggs, poached.
- ✓ Salt and pepper to taste

Instructions:

1. Sauté cauliflower rice and broccoli in olive oil until tender.
2. Top with poached eggs and season with salt and pepper.

Nutritional Information:

230 calories, 10g carbs, 14g protein, 15g fat, 5g fiber.

A low-carb veggie-packed bowl with a protein boost from poached eggs.

Green Spinach and Mushroom Smoothie

Preparation Time: 7 minutes

Serving: 1

Ingredients:

- ✓ 1 cup fresh spinach leaves
- ✓ 1/2 cup cucumber, sliced.
- ✓ 1/4 cup unsweetened almond milk
- ✓ 1/2 avocado
- ✓ 1/2 lime, juiced.

Instructions:

1. Blend spinach, cucumber, almond milk, avocado, and lime juice until smooth.
2. Pour into a glass and enjoy.

Nutritional Information:

180 calories, 8g carbs, 6g protein, 15g fat, 5g fiber.

A refreshing green smoothie for a nutrient-packed start to your day.

Turkey and Cheese Breakfast Quesadilla

Cooking Time: 10 minutes

Serving: 1

Ingredients:

- ✓ 1 low-carb whole-grain tortilla
- ✓ 2 oz turkey slices
- ✓ 1/4 cup shredded cheddar cheese
- ✓ 1/4 cup salsa

Instructions:

1. Place tortilla on a heated pan; add turkey and cheese.
2. Fold in half and cook until cheese melts; serve with salsa.

Nutritional Information:

260 calories, 15g carbs, 20g protein, 12g fat, 4g fiber.

A satisfying and cheesy breakfast quesadilla with a flavorful twist.

CHAPTER 2

WHOLESOME SNACKS

Cucumber and Hummus Bites

Preparation Time: 10 minutes

Serving: 1

Ingredients:

- ✓ 1 cucumber, sliced.
- ✓ 2 tablespoons hummus
- ✓ Cherry tomatoes for garnish
- ✓ Fresh parsley, chopped.

Instructions:

1. Top cucumber slices with hummus.
2. Garnish with cherry tomatoes and parsley.

Nutritional Information:

80 calories, 10g carbs, 3g protein, 4g fat, 2g fiber.

A light and refreshing snack, rich in fiber and healthy fats from hummus.

Almond and Berry Yogurt Parfait

Preparation Time: 5 minutes

Serving: 1

Ingredients:

- ✓ 1/2 cup Greek yogurt
- ✓ 1/4 cup almonds, chopped.
- ✓ 1/4 cup mixed berries
- ✓ 1 teaspoon honey

Instructions:

1. Layer yogurt with almonds and berries.
2. Drizzle with honey before serving.

Nutritional Information:

220 calories, 15g carbs, 12g protein, 14g fat, 4g fiber.

A satisfying and protein-rich parfait with the sweetness of berries.

Baked Zucchini Chips

Preparation Time: 20 minutes

Serving: 2

Ingredients:

- ✓ 2 zucchinis thinly sliced.
- ✓ 1 tablespoon olive oil
- ✓ 1/2 teaspoon garlic powder
- ✓ Salt and pepper to taste

Instructions:

1. Toss zucchini slices in olive oil, garlic powder, salt, and pepper.
2. Bake until crispy; let cool before serving.

Nutritional Information:

120 calories, 10g carbs, 3g protein, 8g fat, 2g fiber.

A crunchy and low-carb alternative to traditional chips.

Tuna and Avocado Lettuce Wraps

Preparation Time: 15 minutes

Serving: 2

Ingredients:

- ✓ 1 can tuna, drained.
- ✓ 1 avocado, mashed.
- ✓ 1 tablespoon Greek yogurt
- ✓ Lettuce leaves for wrapping.

Instructions:

1. Mix tuna with mashed avocado and Greek yogurt.
2. Spoon onto lettuce leaves and wrap.

Nutritional Information:

180 calories, 8g carbs, 20g protein, 10g fat, 4g fiber.

A protein-packed and creamy snack, ideal for a quick and nutritious bite.

Roasted Chickpeas

Preparation Time: 40 minutes

Serving: 4

Ingredients:

- ✓ 2 cans chickpeas drained and rinsed.
- ✓ 1 tablespoon olive oil
- ✓ 1 teaspoon cumin
- ✓ 1/2 teaspoon paprika

Instructions:

1. Toss chickpeas in olive oil, cumin, and paprika.
2. Roast until crispy; cool before serving.

Nutritional Information:

150 calories, 20g carbs, 7g protein, 5g fat, 6g fiber.

A crunchy and fiber-rich alternative to traditional snacks.

Cheese and Veggie Skewers

Preparation Time: 15 minutes

Serving: 2

Ingredients:

- ✓ 1 cup cherry tomatoes
- ✓ 1 cup mozzarella cheese balls
- ✓ 1/2 cup cucumber, sliced.
- ✓ Fresh basil leaves

Instructions:

1. Thread tomatoes, cheese, cucumber, and basil onto skewers.
2. Arrange on a plate before serving.

Nutritional Information:

180 calories, 8g carbs, 12g protein, 10g fat, 2g fiber.

A colorful and flavorful snack, rich in calcium from mozzarella.

Berries and Cottage Cheese Bowl

Preparation Time: 5 minutes

Serving: 1

Ingredients:

- ✓ 1/2 cup cottage cheese
- ✓ 1/2 cup mixed berries
- ✓ 1 tablespoon chopped nuts (e.g., almonds or walnuts)
- ✓ 1 teaspoon honey

Instructions:

1. Combine cottage cheese with berries.
2. Top with chopped nuts and drizzle with honey.

Nutritional Information:

200 calories, 15g carbs, 14g protein, 10g fat, 3g fiber.

A protein-packed and antioxidant-rich bowl for a sweet and satisfying treat.

Celery and Peanut Butter Ants on a Log

Preparation Time: 7 minutes

Serving: 2

Ingredients:

- ✓ 4 celery stalks
- ✓ 4 tablespoons peanut butter
- ✓ Raisins for topping

Instructions:

1. Spread peanut butter on celery.
2. Top with raisins to resemble "ants on a log."

Nutritional Information:

160 calories, 8g carbs, 6g protein, 12g fat, 3g fiber.

A nostalgic and nutritious snack, rich in healthy fats and fiber.

Yogurt and Granola Parfait

Preparation Time: 8 minutes

Serving: 1

Ingredients:

- ✓ 1/2 cup Greek yogurt
- ✓ 1/4 cup low-carb granola
- ✓ 1/4 cup berries
- ✓ 1 tablespoon chia seeds

Instructions:

1. Layer yogurt with granola, berries, and chia seeds.
2. Repeat layers and serve.

Nutritional Information:

240 calories, 20g carbs, 15g protein, 10g fat, 5g fiber.

A crunchy and protein-rich parfait for a wholesome snack.

Egg Salad Lettuce Wraps

Preparation Time: 15 minutes

Serving: 2

Ingredients:

- ✓ 4 hard-boiled eggs, chopped.
- ✓ 2 tablespoons mayonnaise
- ✓ 1 teaspoon Dijon mustard
- ✓ Salt and pepper to taste
- ✓ Lettuce leaves for wrapping.

Instructions:

1. Mix chopped eggs with mayonnaise, mustard, salt, and pepper.
2. Spoon onto lettuce leaves and wrap.

Nutritional Information:

200 calories, 3g carbs, 10g protein, 16g fat, 1g fiber.

A protein-packed and savory snack, perfect for a quick and satisfying bite.

CHAPTER 3

HEARTY SOUPS AND SALADS

Chicken and Vegetable Soup

Cooking Time: 30 minutes

Serving: 4

Ingredients:

- ✓ 1 lb boneless, skinless chicken breasts
- ✓ 4 cups low-sodium chicken broth
- ✓ 2 carrots, diced.
- ✓ 2 celery stalks, chopped
- ✓ 1 onion, diced
- ✓ 2 cloves garlic, minced
- ✓ 1 teaspoon dried thyme
- ✓ Salt and pepper to taste

Instructions:

1. In a pot, combine chicken, broth, carrots, celery, onion, garlic, thyme, salt, and pepper.
2. Simmer until chicken is cooked; shred chicken and return to the pot before serving.

Nutritional Information:

200 calories, 10g carbs, 25g protein, 6g fat, 3g fiber.

Packed with lean protein and veggies, this soup is comforting and diabetes friendly.

Quinoa and Vegetable Salad

Preparation Time: 20 minutes

Serving: 6

Ingredients:

- ✓ 1 cup quinoa, cooked
- ✓ 1 cucumber, diced
- ✓ 1 bell pepper, chopped
- ✓ 1 cup cherry tomatoes, halved
- ✓ 1/4 cup feta cheese, crumbled
- ✓ 2 tablespoons olive oil
- ✓ 1 tablespoon balsamic vinegar
- ✓ Salt and pepper to taste

Instructions:

1. In a bowl, combine quinoa, cucumber, bell pepper, tomatoes, and feta.
2. Drizzle with olive oil and balsamic vinegar, season with salt and pepper, and toss before serving.

Nutritional Information:

250 calories, 30g carbs, 8g protein, 10g fat, 5g fiber.

A nutrient-dense salad with quinoa for sustained energy and a burst of fresh flavors.

Tomato Basil Soup

Cooking Time: 40 minutes

Serving: 4

Ingredients:

- ✓ 6 tomatoes, chopped
- ✓ 1 onion, diced
- ✓ 3 cloves garlic, minced
- ✓ 4 cups low-sodium vegetable broth
- ✓ 1/2 cup fresh basil, chopped
- ✓ 1 teaspoon olive oil
- ✓ Salt and pepper to taste

Instructions:

1. Sauté onion and garlic in olive oil until soft; add tomatoes, broth, basil, salt, and pepper.
2. Simmer until tomatoes are tender; blend until smooth before serving.

Nutritional Information:

120 calories, 15g carbs, 4g protein, 6g fat, 3g fiber.

A low-calorie, antioxidant-rich soup with the classic combination of tomatoes and basil.

Mediterranean Chickpea Salad

Preparation Time: 15 minutes

Serving: 4

Ingredients:

- ✓ 2 cans chickpeas, drained and rinsed
- ✓ 1 cucumber, diced
- ✓ 1 cup cherry tomatoes, halved
- ✓ 1/2 red onion, finely chopped
- ✓ 1/4 cup Kalamata olives, sliced
- ✓ 1/4 cup feta cheese, crumbled
- ✓ 2 tablespoons olive oil
- ✓ 1 tablespoon red wine vinegar
- ✓ Fresh oregano, chopped

Instructions:

1. In a bowl, combine chickpeas, cucumber, tomatoes, red onion, olives, and feta.
2. Drizzle with olive oil and red wine vinegar, sprinkle with oregano, and toss before serving.

Nutritional Information:

280 calories, 30g carbs, 10g protein, 14g fat, 8g fiber.

A Mediterranean-inspired salad with fiber-rich chickpeas and heart-healthy olive oil.

Lentil and Spinach Soup

Cooking Time: 45 minutes

Serving: 6

Ingredients:

- ✓ 1 cup dry green lentils, rinsed
- ✓ 1 onion, diced
- ✓ 2 carrots, sliced
- ✓ 2 celery stalks, chopped
- ✓ 3 cloves garlic, minced
- ✓ 6 cups low-sodium vegetable broth
- ✓ 2 cups fresh spinach, chopped
- ✓ 1 teaspoon cumin
- ✓ Salt and pepper to taste

Instructions:

1. Combine lentils, onion, carrots, celery, garlic, broth, cumin, salt, and pepper in a pot.
2. Simmer until lentils are tender; add spinach and cook until wilted before serving.

Nutritional Information:

220 calories, 35g carbs, 15g protein, 2g fat, 12g fiber.

A high-fiber soup with lentils and spinach for a hearty and nutritious meal.

Kale and Quinoa Salad with Lemon Vinaigrette

Preparation Time: 25 minutes

Serving: 4

Ingredients:

- ✓ 1 cup quinoa, cooked
- ✓ 4 cups kale, chopped
- ✓ 1 cup cherry tomatoes, halved
- ✓ 1/2 cup red onion, thinly sliced
- ✓ 1/4 cup Parmesan cheese, grated
- ✓ 1/4 cup pine nuts, toasted
- ✓ 3 tablespoons olive oil
- ✓ 2 tablespoons lemon juice
- ✓ Salt and pepper to taste

Instructions:

1. In a large bowl, combine quinoa, kale, tomatoes, red onion, Parmesan, and pine nuts.
2. Drizzle with olive oil and lemon juice, season with salt and pepper, and toss before serving.

Nutritional Information:

320 calories, 35g carbs, 12g protein, 16g fat, 5g fiber.

A nutrient-packed salad with kale, quinoa, and a zesty lemon vinaigrette.

Butternut Squash and Apple Soup

Cooking Time: 40 minutes

Serving: 4

Ingredients:

- ✓ 1 butternut squash, peeled and diced
- ✓ 2 apples, peeled and chopped
- ✓ 1 onion, diced
- ✓ 2 cloves garlic, minced
- ✓ 4 cups low-sodium vegetable broth
- ✓ 1 teaspoon curry powder
- ✓ 1/2 teaspoon nutmeg
- ✓ Salt and pepper to taste

Instructions:

1. In a pot, combine butternut squash, apples, onion, garlic, broth, curry powder, nutmeg, salt, and pepper.
2. Simmer until squash and apples are tender; blend until smooth before serving.

Nutritional Information:

A comforting soup with the sweetness of butternut squash and apples.

Shrimp and Avocado Salad

Preparation Time: 15 minutes

Serving: 2

Ingredients:

- ✓ 1 lb shrimp, cooked and peeled
- ✓ 2 avocados, diced
- ✓ 1 cup cherry tomatoes, halved
- ✓ 1/4 cup red onion, finely chopped
- ✓ 1/4 cup cilantro, chopped
- ✓ 2 tablespoons olive oil
- ✓ 1 tablespoon lime juice
- ✓ Salt and pepper to taste

Instructions:

1. In a bowl, combine shrimp, avocados, tomatoes, red onion, and cilantro.
2. Drizzle with olive oil and lime juice, season with salt and pepper, and toss before serving.

Nutritional Information:

290 calories, 15g carbs, 25g protein, 18g fat, 8g fiber.

A protein-rich salad with the goodness of shrimp and creamy avocado.

Minestrone Soup

Cooking Time: 35 minutes

Serving: 6

Ingredients:

- ✓ 1 cup whole wheat pasta, cooked
- ✓ 1 can kidney beans, drained and rinsed
- ✓ 1 cup zucchini, diced
- ✓ 1 cup carrots, sliced
- ✓ 1 cup celery, chopped
- ✓ 1 onion, diced
- ✓ 3 cloves garlic, minced
- ✓ 4 cups low-sodium vegetable broth
- ✓ 1 can diced tomatoes
- ✓ 1 teaspoon dried oregano
- ✓ Salt and pepper to taste

Instructions:

1. In a pot, combine pasta, beans, zucchini, carrots, celery, onion, garlic, broth, tomatoes, oregano, salt, and pepper.
2. Simmer until vegetables are tender before serving.

Nutritional Information:

250 calories, 45g carbs, 12g protein, 2g fat, 10g fiber.

A hearty and high-fiber soup with a variety of vegetables and whole wheat pasta.

Greek Salad with Grilled Chicken

Preparation Time: 30 minutes

Serving: 4

Ingredients:

- ✓ 1 lb chicken breasts, grilled and sliced
- ✓ 4 cups romaine lettuce, chopped
- ✓ 1 cucumber, diced
- ✓ 1 cup cherry tomatoes, halved
- ✓ 1/2 cup red onion, thinly sliced
- ✓ 1/4 cup Kalamata olives, sliced
- ✓ 1/4 cup feta cheese, crumbled
- ✓ 2 tablespoons olive oil
- ✓ 1 tablespoon red wine vinegar
- ✓ 1 teaspoon dried oregano
- ✓ Salt and pepper to taste

Instructions:

1. In a large bowl, combine grilled chicken, lettuce, cucumber, tomatoes, red onion, olives, and feta.
2. Drizzle with olive oil and red wine vinegar, sprinkle with oregano, season with salt and pepper, and toss before serving.

Nutritional Information:

320 calories, 15g carbs, 30g protein, 18g fat, 5g fiber.

A protein-packed salad with grilled chicken and the flavors of a classic Greek salad.

Broccoli and Cheddar Soup

Cooking Time: 25 minutes

Serving: 4

Ingredients:

- ✓ 2 cups broccoli florets
- ✓ 1 onion, diced
- ✓ 2 carrots, sliced
- ✓ 2 cups low-sodium vegetable broth
- ✓ 1 cup sharp cheddar cheese, shredded
- ✓ 1 cup unsweetened almond milk
- ✓ 2 tablespoons whole wheat flour
- ✓ 1 teaspoon olive oil
- ✓ Salt and pepper to taste

Instructions:

1. Sauté onion in olive oil until soft; add broccoli, carrots, and flour.
2. Pour in broth and almond milk; simmer until veggies are tender. Stir in cheddar until melted before serving.

Nutritional Information:

240 calories, 20g carbs, 12g protein, 14g fat, 6g fiber.

A creamy and cheesy soup with the goodness of broccoli for a comforting meal.

Spinach and Strawberry Salad with Balsamic Vinaigrette

Preparation Time: 15 minutes

Serving: 4

Ingredients:

- ✓ 6 cups baby spinach
- ✓ 1 cup strawberries, sliced
- ✓ 1/4 cup red onion, thinly sliced
- ✓ 1/4 cup goat cheese, crumbled
- ✓ 1/4 cup balsamic vinegar
- ✓ 2 tablespoons olive oil
- ✓ 1 tablespoon honey
- ✓ Salt and pepper to taste

Instructions:

1. In a large bowl, combine spinach, strawberries, red onion, and goat cheese.
2. Whisk together balsamic vinegar, olive oil, honey, salt, and pepper. Drizzle over the salad and toss before serving.

Nutritional Information:

180 calories, 15g carbs, 6g protein, 12g fat, 4g fiber.

A refreshing salad with the sweetness of strawberries and the tanginess of balsamic vinaigrette.

Cabbage and Sausage Soup

Cooking Time: 35 minutes

Serving: 6

Ingredients:

- ✓ 1 lb turkey sausage, sliced
- ✓ 1 small cabbage, shredded
- ✓ 2 carrots, diced
- ✓ 2 potatoes, peeled and diced
- ✓ 1 onion, diced
- ✓ 4 cups low-sodium chicken broth
- ✓ 1 teaspoon caraway seeds
- ✓ Salt and pepper to taste

Instructions:

1. In a pot, brown sausage; add cabbage, carrots, potatoes, onion, broth, caraway seeds, salt, and pepper.
2. Simmer until vegetables are tender before serving.

Nutritional Information:

280 calories, 30g carbs, 15g protein, 10g fat, 8g fiber.

A hearty and filling soup with the savory goodness of turkey sausage and cabbage.

Caesar Salad with Grilled Salmon

Preparation Time: 20 minutes

Serving: 4

Ingredients:

- ✓ 1 lb salmon fillets, grilled
- ✓ 6 cups romaine lettuce, chopped
- ✓ 1 cup cherry tomatoes, halved
- ✓ 1/2 cup croutons (whole wheat for a healthier option)
- ✓ 1/4 cup Parmesan cheese, shaved
- ✓ 1/4 cup Caesar dressing (low-fat)

Instructions:

1. In a large bowl, combine grilled salmon, romaine lettuce, tomatoes, croutons, and Parmesan.
2. Drizzle with Caesar dressing and toss before serving.

Nutritional Information:

320 calories, 20g carbs, 30g protein, 15g fat, 5g fiber.

A protein-packed Caesar salad featuring grilled salmon for a satisfying and nutritious meal.

Sweet Potato and Black Bean Chili

Cooking Time: 40 minutes

Serving: 6

Ingredients:

- ✓ 2 sweet potatoes, peeled and diced
- ✓ 2 cans black beans, drained and rinsed
- ✓ 1 onion, diced
- ✓ 3 cloves garlic, minced
- ✓ 1 can diced tomatoes
- ✓ 4 cups low-sodium vegetable broth
- ✓ 2 teaspoons chili powder
- ✓ 1 teaspoon cumin
- ✓ Salt and pepper to taste

Instructions:

1. In a pot, combine sweet potatoes, black beans, onion, garlic, tomatoes, broth, chili powder, cumin, salt, and pepper.
2. Simmer until sweet potatoes are tender before serving.

Nutritional Information:

260 calories, 45g carbs, 10g protein, 1g fat, 12g fiber.

A fiber-rich and flavorful chili featuring sweet potatoes and black beans.

Asian Chicken Salad

Preparation Time: 25 minutes

Serving: 4

Ingredients:

- ✓ 1 lb chicken breasts, grilled and sliced.
- ✓ 6 cups Napa cabbage, shredded.
- ✓ 1 cup snow peas, sliced.
- ✓ 1/2 cup shredded carrots
- ✓ 1/4 cup sliced almonds, toasted.
- ✓ 2 tablespoons sesame oil
- ✓ 2 tablespoons soy sauce (low sodium)
- ✓ 1 tablespoon rice vinegar
- ✓ 1 teaspoon honey

Instructions:

1. In a large bowl, combine grilled chicken, Napa cabbage, snow peas, carrots, and almonds.
2. Whisk together sesame oil, soy sauce, rice vinegar, and honey. Drizzle over the salad and toss before serving.

Nutritional Information:

290 calories, 15g carbs, 25g protein, 15g fat, 6g fiber.

An Asian-inspired salad with grilled chicken, crunchy vegetables, and a flavorful sesame dressing.

Vegetarian Lentil Soup

Cooking Time: 45 minutes

Serving: 6

Ingredients:

- ✓ 1 cup dry brown lentils, rinsed
- ✓ 2 carrots, diced
- ✓ 2 celery stalks, chopped
- ✓ 1 onion, diced
- ✓ 3 cloves garlic, minced
- ✓ 6 cups low-sodium vegetable broth
- ✓ 1 can diced tomatoes
- ✓ 1 teaspoon ground cumin
- ✓ 1/2 teaspoon smoked paprika
- ✓ Salt and pepper to taste

Instructions:

1. Combine lentils, carrots, celery, onion, garlic, broth, tomatoes, cumin, paprika, salt, and pepper in a pot.
2. Simmer until lentils are tender before serving.

Nutritional Information:

240 calories, 40g carbs, 15g protein, 1g fat, 10g fiber.

A protein-packed and fiber-rich lentil soup for a satisfying and nutritious meal.

Caprese Salad with Balsamic Glaze

Preparation Time: 15 minutes

Serving: 4

Ingredients:

- ✓ 4 large tomatoes, sliced
- ✓ 1 lb fresh mozzarella cheese, sliced
- ✓ Fresh basil leaves
- ✓ 2 tablespoons balsamic glaze
- ✓ 2 tablespoons extra-virgin olive oil
- ✓ Salt and pepper to taste

Instructions:

1. Arrange tomato and mozzarella slices on a plate, alternating with basil leaves.
2. Drizzle with balsamic glaze and olive oil, season with salt and pepper, and serve.

Nutritional Information:

320 calories, 10g carbs, 20g protein, 25g fat, 3g fiber.

A classic Caprese salad with the added richness of balsamic glaze for a delightful and light meal.

Cauliflower and Leek Soup

Cooking Time: 30 minutes

Serving: 4

Ingredients:

- ✓ 1 cauliflower head, chopped
- ✓ 2 leeks, sliced
- ✓ 2 potatoes, peeled and diced
- ✓ 1 onion, diced
- ✓ 4 cups low-sodium vegetable broth
- ✓ 2 tablespoons olive oil
- ✓ 1 teaspoon dried thyme
- ✓ Salt and pepper to taste

Instructions:

1. Sauté leeks and onion in olive oil until soft; add cauliflower, potatoes, broth, thyme, salt, and pepper.
2. Simmer until vegetables are tender; blend until smooth before serving.

Nutritional Information:

180 calories, 25g carbs, 5g protein, 8g fat, 5g fiber.

A velvety and low-calorie soup featuring cauliflower and leeks for a comforting option.

Tuna Nicoise Salad

Preparation Time: 20 minutes

Serving: 4

Ingredients:

- ✓ 2 cans tuna, drained
- ✓ 6 cups mixed salad greens
- ✓ 4 hard-boiled eggs, sliced
- ✓ 1 cup cherry tomatoes, halved
- ✓ 1/2 cup green beans, blanched
- ✓ 1/4 cup Kalamata olives, sliced
- ✓ 2 tablespoons Dijon mustard vinaigrette
- ✓ Salt and pepper to taste

Instructions:

1. Arrange salad greens on plates; top with tuna, eggs, tomatoes, green beans, and olives.
2. Drizzle with Dijon mustard vinaigrette, season with salt and pepper, and serve.

Nutritional Information:

280 calories, 15g carbs, 30g protein, 12g fat, 6g fiber.

A protein-packed and vibrant tuna salad with a variety of textures and flavors.

CHAPTER 4

FLAVORFUL MAIN COURSES

Grilled Lemon Herb Chicken

Cooking Time: 25 minutes

Serving: 4

Ingredients:

- ✓ 4 boneless, skinless chicken breasts
- ✓ 2 lemons, juiced.
- ✓ 2 tablespoons olive oil
- ✓ 2 teaspoons dried thyme
- ✓ 1 teaspoon garlic powder
- ✓ Salt and pepper to taste

Instructions:

1. In a bowl, mix lemon juice, olive oil, thyme, garlic powder, salt, and pepper.
2. Marinate chicken in the mixture, then grill until cooked through.

Nutritional Information:

220 calories, 1g carbs, 30g protein, 10g fat, 0g fiber.

A flavorful and low-carb grilled chicken dish, rich in lean protein and zesty herbs.

Salmon with Dill Sauce

Cooking Time: 20 minutes

Serving: 4

Ingredients:

- ✓ 4 salmon fillets
- ✓ 1/4 cup Greek yogurt
- ✓ 2 tablespoons fresh dill, chopped
- ✓ 1 tablespoon Dijon mustard
- ✓ 1 lemon, sliced
- ✓ Salt and pepper to taste

Instructions:

1. Season salmon with salt and pepper, then bake until flaky.
2. Mix Greek yogurt, dill, and Dijon for the sauce. Serve salmon with a dollop of sauce and lemon slices.

Nutritional Information:

280 calories, 2g carbs, 25g protein, 18g fat, 0g fiber.

A heart-healthy salmon dish with a refreshing dill sauce, providing omega-3 fatty acids.

Turkey and Vegetable Stir-Fry

Cooking Time: 20 minutes

Serving: 4

Ingredients:

- ✓ 1 lb ground turkey
- ✓ 2 cups broccoli florets
- ✓ 1 bell pepper, sliced
- ✓ 1 cup snap peas
- ✓ 2 tablespoons low-sodium soy sauce
- ✓ 1 tablespoon sesame oil
- ✓ 1 teaspoon ginger, minced
- ✓ 2 cloves garlic, minced
- ✓ 1 tablespoon olive oil

Instructions:

1. In a pan, brown turkey in olive oil; add broccoli, bell pepper, snap peas, ginger, and garlic.
2. Stir in soy sauce and sesame oil until veggies are tender.

Nutritional Information:

280 calories, 10g carbs, 25g protein, 15g fat, 4g fiber.

A quick and savory turkey stir-fry loaded with colorful vegetables and Asian-inspired flavors.

Eggplant and Chickpea Curry

Cooking Time: 30 minutes

Serving: 4

Ingredients:

- ✓ 1 large eggplant, diced
- ✓ 1 can chickpeas, drained and rinsed
- ✓ 1 onion, diced
- ✓ 2 tomatoes, chopped
- ✓ 1/4 cup curry powder
- ✓ 1 teaspoon cumin
- ✓ 1 teaspoon turmeric
- ✓ 1 tablespoon olive oil
- ✓ Salt and pepper to taste

Instructions:

1. Sauté onion in olive oil; add eggplant, chickpeas, tomatoes, curry powder, cumin, turmeric, salt, and pepper.
2. Simmer until eggplant is tender. Serve over cauliflower rice.

Nutritional Information:

240 calories, 35g carbs, 9g protein, 10g fat, 10g fiber.

A fiber-rich and flavorful vegetarian curry, perfect for a satisfying and healthy meal.

Baked Cod with Mediterranean Salsa

Cooking Time: 20 minutes

Serving: 4

Ingredients:

- ✓ 4 cod fillets
- ✓ 1 cup cherry tomatoes, halved
- ✓ 1/2 cup Kalamata olives, sliced
- ✓ 1/4 cup red onion, finely chopped
- ✓ 2 tablespoons fresh parsley, chopped
- ✓ 1 tablespoon olive oil
- ✓ 1 lemon, juiced
- ✓ Salt and pepper to taste

Instructions:

1. Season cod with salt and pepper, bake until opaque.
2. Mix tomatoes, olives, red onion, parsley, olive oil, and lemon juice for salsa. Top cod with salsa before serving.

Nutritional Information:

220 calories, 5g carbs, 30g protein, 9g fat, 2g fiber.

A light and vibrant cod dish with a Mediterranean twist, offering a burst of fresh flavors.

Stuffed Bell Peppers with Turkey and Quinoa

Cooking Time: 40 minutes

Serving: 4

Ingredients:

- ✓ 4 bell peppers, halved and seeds removed
- ✓ 1 lb ground turkey
- ✓ 1 cup cooked quinoa
- ✓ 1 can black beans, drained and rinsed
- ✓ 1 cup corn kernels
- ✓ 1 cup salsa
- ✓ 1 teaspoon cumin
- ✓ 1/2 teaspoon chili powder
- ✓ Salt and pepper to taste

Instructions:

1. Preheat oven and bake bell peppers until slightly tender.
2. In a skillet, brown turkey; add quinoa, black beans, corn, salsa, cumin, chili powder, salt, and pepper. Stuff bell peppers with the mixture and bake until heated through.

Nutritional Information:

320 calories, 35g carbs, 25g protein, 10g fat, 8g fiber.

A nutritious and colorful dish featuring lean turkey, quinoa, and a variety of veggies for a balanced meal.

Lemon Garlic Shrimp with Zucchini Noodles

Cooking Time: 15 minutes

Serving: 2

Ingredients:

- ✓ 1 lb shrimp, peeled and deveined
- ✓ 3 zucchinis, spiralized
- ✓ 2 tablespoons olive oil
- ✓ 3 cloves garlic, minced
- ✓ 1 lemon, juiced and zested
- ✓ 1/4 teaspoon red pepper flakes
- ✓ Salt and pepper to taste

Instructions:

1. Sauté shrimp in olive oil with garlic, lemon juice, zest, red pepper flakes, salt, and pepper.
2. Add zucchini noodles and cook until tender. Serve immediately.

Nutritional Information:

280 calories, 10g carbs, 30g protein, 14g fat, 3g fiber.

A light and zesty shrimp dish with zucchini noodles, offering a low-carb alternative to traditional pasta.

Sesame Ginger Tofu Stir-Fry

Cooking Time: 25 minutes

Serving: 4

Ingredients:

- ✓ 1 lb firm tofu, cubed
- ✓ 2 cups broccoli florets
- ✓ 1 bell pepper, sliced
- ✓ 1 cup snow peas
- ✓ 2 tablespoons low-sodium soy sauce
- ✓ 1 tablespoon sesame oil
- ✓ 1 tablespoon rice vinegar
- ✓ 1 tablespoon fresh ginger, grated
- ✓ 1 tablespoon olive oil

Instructions:

1. Press tofu to remove excess water; stir-fry tofu, broccoli, bell pepper, and snow peas in olive oil.
2. Whisk together soy sauce, sesame oil, rice vinegar, and ginger. Drizzle over stir-fry before serving.

Nutritional Information:

260 calories, 15g carbs, 15g protein, 15g fat, 4g fiber.

A vegetarian stir-fry with tofu and crisp vegetables, infused with a savory sesame ginger sauce.

Cauliflower Crust Pizza

Cooking Time: 30 minutes

Serving: 2

Ingredients:

- ✓ 1 cauliflower head, riced
- ✓ 1/2 cup mozzarella cheese, shredded
- ✓ 1 egg
- ✓ 1/4 cup tomato sauce (no sugar added)
- ✓ 1/2 cup cherry tomatoes, sliced
- ✓ 1/4 cup olives, sliced
- ✓ 1/4 cup fresh basil, chopped
- ✓ Salt and pepper to taste

Instructions:

1. Mix cauliflower rice, mozzarella, and egg; press into a crust and bake until golden.
2. Spread tomato sauce on the crust, top with tomatoes, olives, basil, salt, and pepper. Bake until cheese is melted.

Nutritional Information:

230 calories, 20g carbs, 12g protein, 12g fat, 8g fiber.

A guilt-free pizza with a cauliflower crust, providing a tasty and low-carb alternative.

Beef and Vegetable Skewers

Cooking Time: 15 minutes

Serving: 4

Ingredients:

- ✓ 1 lb beef sirloin, cut into cubes
- ✓ 2 bell peppers, cut into chunks
- ✓ 1 red onion, cut into chunks
- ✓ 1 zucchini, sliced
- ✓ 2 tablespoons olive oil
- ✓ 1 teaspoon smoked paprika
- ✓ 1 teaspoon garlic powder
- ✓ Salt and pepper to taste

Instructions:

1. Thread beef, peppers, onion, and zucchini onto skewers.
2. Mix olive oil, smoked paprika, garlic powder, salt, and pepper. Brush over skewers and grill until beef is cooked to desired doneness.

Nutritional Information:

300 calories, 10g carbs, 25g protein, 18g fat, 4g fiber.

Flavorful beef skewers with a variety of veggies, offering a balanced and satisfying main course.

Mushroom and Spinach Stuffed Chicken

Cooking Time: 30 minutes

Serving: 4

Ingredients:

- ✓ 4 boneless, skinless chicken breasts
- ✓ 2 cups mushrooms, chopped
- ✓ 2 cups fresh spinach, chopped
- ✓ 1/2 cup feta cheese, crumbled
- ✓ 1 tablespoon olive oil
- ✓ 2 cloves garlic, minced
- ✓ 1 teaspoon dried oregano
- ✓ Salt and pepper to taste

Instructions:

1. Sauté mushrooms and spinach in olive oil with garlic until wilted; stir in feta, oregano, salt, and pepper.
2. Cut a pocket into each chicken breast, stuff with the mushroom-spinach mixture, and bake until chicken is cooked through.

Nutritional Information:

250 calories, 4g carbs, 30g protein, 12g fat, 2g fiber.

A savory and nutrient-packed dish with chicken breasts stuffed with a flavorful mushroom and spinach filling.

Vegetarian Zucchini Lasagna

Cooking Time: 45 minutes

Serving: 6

Ingredients:

- ✓ 3 large zucchinis, sliced lengthwise
- ✓ 2 cups ricotta cheese
- ✓ 1 cup mozzarella cheese, shredded
- ✓ 1 cup spinach, chopped
- ✓ 1 can crushed tomatoes (no sugar added)
- ✓ 2 cloves garlic, minced
- ✓ 1 teaspoon dried basil
- ✓ Salt and pepper to taste

Instructions:

1. Mix ricotta, mozzarella, spinach, garlic, basil, salt, and pepper.
2. Layer zucchini slices with ricotta mixture and crushed tomatoes, repeat, and bake until bubbly and golden.

Nutritional Information:

220 calories, 12g carbs, 15g protein, 14g fat, 4g fiber.

A low-carb twist on classic lasagna, featuring zucchini layers and a rich, vegetarian ricotta filling.

Lemon Herb Baked Cod

Cooking Time: 20 minutes

Serving: 4

Ingredients:

- ✓ 4 cod fillets
- ✓ 1/4 cup fresh lemon juice
- ✓ 2 tablespoons olive oil
- ✓ 1 tablespoon fresh parsley, chopped.
- ✓ 1 teaspoon dried dill
- ✓ 1 teaspoon garlic powder
- ✓ Salt and pepper to taste

Instructions:

1. Marinate cod in lemon juice, olive oil, parsley, dill, garlic powder, salt, and pepper.
2. Bake until cod is flaky and infused with citrus and herb flavors.

Nutritional Information:

200 calories, 1g carbs, 30g protein, 10g fat, 0g fiber.

A light and refreshing baked cod dish with a zesty lemon-herb marinade.

Cajun Shrimp and Cauliflower Rice

Cooking Time: 25 minutes

Serving: 4

Ingredients:

- ✓ 1 lb shrimp, peeled and deveined
- ✓ 1 head cauliflower, riced
- ✓ 1 bell pepper, diced
- ✓ 1 onion, diced
- ✓ 2 cloves garlic, minced
- ✓ 2 tablespoons Cajun seasoning
- ✓ 1 tablespoon olive oil
- ✓ Salt and pepper to taste

Instructions:

1. Sauté shrimp, bell pepper, onion, and garlic in olive oil with Cajun seasoning.
2. Stir in cauliflower rice until cooked through, creating a flavorful and low-carb shrimp stir-fry.

Nutritional Information:

240 calories, 10g carbs, 25g protein, 12g fat, 4g fiber.

A spicy and satisfying Cajun shrimp dish served over cauliflower rice for a carb-conscious alternative.

Quinoa and Vegetable Stuffed Peppers

Cooking Time: 40 minutes

Serving: 4

Ingredients:

- ✓ 4 bell peppers, halved and seeds removed
- ✓ 1 cup cooked quinoa
- ✓ 1 can black beans, drained and rinsed
- ✓ 1 cup corn kernels
- ✓ 1 cup cherry tomatoes, diced
- ✓ 1/2 cup shredded cheddar cheese
- ✓ 1 teaspoon cumin
- ✓ 1/2 teaspoon chili powder
- ✓ Salt and pepper to taste

Instructions:

1. Preheat oven and bake bell peppers until slightly tender.
2. Mix quinoa, black beans, corn, tomatoes, cheese, cumin, chili powder, salt, and pepper; stuff bell peppers and bake until golden.

Nutritional Information:

290 calories, 40g carbs, 12g protein, 10g fat, 8g fiber.

A colorful and nutrient-packed dish with quinoa and vegetables stuffed in bell peppers.

Sesame Teriyaki Chicken Stir-Fry

Cooking Time: 25 minutes

Serving: 4

Ingredients:

- ✓ 1 lb boneless, skinless chicken thighs, sliced
- ✓ 2 cups broccoli florets
- ✓ 1 bell pepper, sliced
- ✓ 1 cup snap peas
- ✓ 1/4 cup low-sodium teriyaki sauce
- ✓ 2 tablespoons sesame oil
- ✓ 2 tablespoons soy sauce (low-sodium)
- ✓ 1 tablespoon honey
- ✓ 1 tablespoon ginger, minced

Instructions:

1. Stir-fry chicken, broccoli, bell pepper, and snap peas in sesame oil until chicken is cooked.
2. Whisk together teriyaki sauce, soy sauce, honey, and ginger; drizzle over stir-fry and toss before serving.

Nutritional Information:

280 calories, 15g carbs, 25g protein, 14g fat, 4g fiber.

A flavorful and satisfying teriyaki chicken stir-fry with a variety of crisp vegetables.

Cauliflower and Chickpea Curry

Cooking Time: 30 minutes

Serving: 4

Ingredients:

- ✓ 1 head cauliflower, chopped
- ✓ 1 can chickpeas, drained and rinsed
- ✓ 1 onion, diced
- ✓ 2 tomatoes, chopped
- ✓ 1/4 cup curry powder
- ✓ 1 teaspoon cumin
- ✓ 1 teaspoon turmeric
- ✓ 1 tablespoon olive oil
- ✓ Salt and pepper to taste

Instructions:

1. Sauté onion in olive oil; add cauliflower, chickpeas, tomatoes, curry powder, cumin, turmeric, salt, and pepper.
2. Simmer until cauliflower is tender. Serve over cauliflower rice.

Nutritional Information:

240 calories, 35g carbs, 9g protein, 10g fat, 10g fiber.

A fiber-rich and flavorful vegetarian curry featuring cauliflower and protein-packed chickpeas.

Mediterranean Turkey Skillet

Cooking Time: 30 minutes

Serving: 4

Ingredients:

- ✓ 1 lb ground turkey
- ✓ 1 cup cherry tomatoes, halved
- ✓ 1/2 cup Kalamata olives, sliced
- ✓ 1/4 cup feta cheese, crumbled
- ✓ 1/4 cup fresh basil, chopped
- ✓ 2 tablespoons olive oil
- ✓ 2 cloves garlic, minced
- ✓ 1 teaspoon dried oregano
- ✓ Salt and pepper to taste

Instructions:

1. Brown turkey in olive oil with garlic; add tomatoes, olives, feta, basil, oregano, salt, and pepper.
2. Simmer until tomatoes are softened. Serve over zucchini noodles or cauliflower rice.

Nutritional Information:

290 calories, 8g carbs, 25g protein, 18g fat, 2g fiber.

A Mediterranean-inspired turkey skillet with vibrant flavors and wholesome ingredients.

Spaghetti Squash with Turkey Bolognese

Cooking Time: 40 minutes

Serving: 4

Ingredients:

- ✓ 1 spaghetti squash, halved and seeded
- ✓ 1 lb ground turkey
- ✓ 1 can crushed tomatoes (no sugar added)
- ✓ 1 onion, diced
- ✓ 2 cloves garlic, minced
- ✓ 1 teaspoon dried oregano
- ✓ 1 teaspoon dried basil
- ✓ 1 tablespoon olive oil
- ✓ Salt and pepper to taste

Instructions:

1. Roast spaghetti squash until tender; shred with a fork.
2. In a pan, brown turkey in olive oil; add onion, garlic, crushed tomatoes, oregano, basil, salt, and pepper. Simmer until flavors meld. Serve over spaghetti squash.

Nutritional Information:

270 calories, 20g carbs, 25g protein, 14g fat, 5g fiber.

A satisfying and low-carb alternative to traditional spaghetti, featuring spaghetti squash and a savory turkey bolognese.

Lemon Garlic Asparagus and Shrimp

Cooking Time: 20 minutes

Serving: 4

Ingredients:

- ✓ 1 lb shrimp, peeled and deveined
- ✓ 1 lb asparagus, trimmed
- ✓ 2 tablespoons olive oil
- ✓ 3 cloves garlic, minced
- ✓ 1 lemon, zested and juiced
- ✓ 1 teaspoon dried thyme
- ✓ Salt and pepper to taste

Instructions:

1. Sauté shrimp and asparagus in olive oil with garlic until shrimp are pink and asparagus is tender.
2. Sprinkle with lemon zest, lemon juice, thyme, salt, and pepper. Toss before serving.

Nutritional Information:

230 calories, 8g carbs, 25g protein, 12g fat, 4g fiber.

A light and flavorful dish featuring lemon-garlic shrimp paired with vibrant asparagus.

CHAPTER 5

SATISFYING SIDES

Garlic Parmesan Roasted Brussels Sprouts

Cooking Time: 25 minutes

Serving: 4

Ingredients:

- ✓ 1 lb Brussels sprouts, halved
- ✓ 2 tablespoons olive oil
- ✓ 3 cloves garlic, minced
- ✓ 1/4 cup grated Parmesan cheese
- ✓ Salt and pepper to taste

Instructions:

1. Toss Brussels sprouts with olive oil and garlic; roast until crispy.
2. Sprinkle with Parmesan, salt, and pepper before serving.

Nutritional Information:

120 calories, 10g carbs, 5g protein, 8g fat, 4g fiber.

A flavorful and low-carb side dish, featuring roasted Brussels sprouts with a hint of garlic and Parmesan for a satisfying crunch.

Cauliflower Mash with Garlic and Chives

Cooking Time: 20 minutes

Serving: 4

Ingredients:

- ✓ 1 head cauliflower, chopped
- ✓ 2 cloves garlic, minced
- ✓ 2 tablespoons unsalted butter
- ✓ 2 tablespoons fresh chives, chopped
- ✓ Salt and pepper to taste

Instructions:

1. Steam cauliflower until tender; blend with garlic, butter, chives, salt, and pepper until smooth.
2. Serve as a creamy and low-carb alternative to mashed potatoes.

Nutritional Information:

80 calories, 6g carbs, 3g protein, 6g fat, 3g fiber.

A satisfying cauliflower mash infused with garlic and chives, providing a tasty and diabetes-friendly side.

Sautéed Lemon Garlic Spinach

Cooking Time: 10 minutes

Serving: 4

Ingredients:

- ✓ 1 lb fresh spinach
- ✓ 2 tablespoons olive oil
- ✓ 3 cloves garlic, minced
- ✓ 1 lemon, zested and juiced
- ✓ Salt and pepper to taste

Instructions:

1. Sauté spinach in olive oil with garlic until wilted.
2. Sprinkle with lemon zest and juice, season with salt and pepper, and serve as a vibrant and low-carb side.

Nutritional Information:

60 calories, 4g carbs, 3g protein, 4g fat, 2g fiber.

A quick and refreshing side of lemon garlic spinach, adding a burst of flavor and essential nutrients to your meal.

Rosemary Roasted Sweet Potatoes

Cooking Time: 30 minutes

Serving: 4

Ingredients:

- ✓ 2 large sweet potatoes, diced
- ✓ 2 tablespoons olive oil
- ✓ 1 tablespoon fresh rosemary, chopped
- ✓ Salt and pepper to taste

Instructions:

1. Toss sweet potatoes with olive oil and rosemary; roast until golden.
2. Season with salt and pepper, offering a savory and fiber-rich alternative to traditional potatoes.

Nutritional Information:

140 calories, 20g carbs, 2g protein, 6g fat, 4g fiber.

A fragrant and diabetes-friendly side of rosemary roasted sweet potatoes, providing a delightful twist to a classic dish.

Green Bean Almondine

Cooking Time: 15 minutes

Serving: 4

Ingredients:

- ✓ 1 lb green beans, trimmed
- ✓ 2 tablespoons unsalted butter
- ✓ 1/4 cup sliced almonds
- ✓ 1 lemon, zested
- ✓ Salt and pepper to taste

Instructions:

1. Blanch green beans; sauté in butter with almonds until crisp-tender.
2. Sprinkle with lemon zest, salt, and pepper, creating a flavorful and nutritious green bean side.

Nutritional Information:

90 calories, 8g carbs, 2g protein, 6g fat, 4g fiber.

An elegant green bean almondine side dish, combining the crunch of almonds with the freshness of lemon.

Grilled Asparagus with Balsamic Glaze

Cooking Time: 15 minutes

Serving: 4

Ingredients:

- ✓ 1 lb asparagus, trimmed
- ✓ 2 tablespoons olive oil
- ✓ 2 tablespoons balsamic glaze
- ✓ Salt and pepper to taste

Instructions:

1. Toss asparagus with olive oil; grill until slightly charred.
2. Drizzle with balsamic glaze, season with salt and pepper, offering a simple and flavorful grilled side.

Nutritional Information:

70 calories, 8g carbs, 2g protein, 4g fat, 3g fiber.

A char-grilled asparagus side with a drizzle of balsamic glaze, elevating the flavors of this nutrient-rich vegetable.

Mushroom and Thyme Quinoa

Cooking Time: 20 minutes

Serving: 4

Ingredients:

- ✓ 1 cup quinoa, cooked
- ✓ 1 lb mushrooms, sliced
- ✓ 2 tablespoons olive oil
- ✓ 1 tablespoon fresh thyme, chopped
- ✓ Salt and pepper to taste

Instructions:

1. Sauté mushrooms in olive oil with thyme; toss with cooked quinoa.
2. Season with salt and pepper, creating a hearty and protein-packed quinoa side with earthy mushroom flavors.

Nutritional Information:

220 calories, 30g carbs, 8g protein, 8g fat, 4g fiber.

A savory quinoa side featuring mushrooms and thyme, offering a satisfying and nutritious addition to your meal.

Baked Parmesan Zucchini Fries

Cooking Time: 20 minutes

Serving: 4

Ingredients:

- ✓ 2 zucchinis, cut into fries
- ✓ 1/2 cup grated Parmesan cheese
- ✓ 1/4 cup almond flour
- ✓ 1 teaspoon garlic powder
- ✓ 1 teaspoon dried oregano
- ✓ Salt and pepper to taste

Instructions:

1. Mix Parmesan, almond flour, garlic powder, oregano, salt, and pepper.
2. Coat zucchini fries in the mixture; bake until golden and crispy, providing a low-carb alternative to traditional fries.

Nutritional Information:

110 calories, 8g carbs, 6g protein, 7g fat, 2g fiber.

Baked Parmesan zucchini fries, a guilt-free and flavorful side, perfect for satisfying cravings without the excess carbs.

Tomato Avocado Salad

Cooking Time: 10 minutes

Serving: 4

Ingredients:

- ✓ 2 cups cherry tomatoes, halved
- ✓ 2 avocados, diced
- ✓ 1/4 cup red onion, finely chopped
- ✓ 2 tablespoons fresh basil, chopped
- ✓ 1 tablespoon balsamic vinegar
- ✓ 1 tablespoon olive oil
- ✓ Salt and pepper to taste

Instructions:

1. Combine tomatoes, avocados, red onion, and basil; drizzle with balsamic vinegar and olive oil.
2. Season with salt and pepper, creating a refreshing and nutrient-packed tomato avocado salad.

Nutritional Information: 180 calories, 12g carbs, 3g protein, 15g fat, 7g fiber.

A vibrant and flavorful tomato avocado salad, offering a dose of healthy fats and fresh produce to complement any meal.

Lemon Herb Cauliflower Rice

Cooking Time: 15 minutes

Serving: 4

Ingredients:

- ✓ 1 head cauliflower, riced
- ✓ 2 tablespoons olive oil
- ✓ 1 lemon, zested and juiced
- ✓ 1 tablespoon fresh parsley, chopped
- ✓ 1 teaspoon dried thyme
- ✓ Salt and pepper to taste

Instructions:

1. Sauté cauliflower rice in olive oil until tender; mix in lemon zest, lemon juice, parsley, thyme, salt, and pepper.
2. Serve as a light and citrusy alternative to traditional rice, adding zest and flavor to your meal.

Nutritional Information:

70 calories, 8g carbs, 2g protein, 4g fat, 3g fiber.

Info: Lemon herb cauliflower rice, a low-carb and flavorful side, providing a refreshing twist to your favorite rice dishes.

CHAPTER 6

28 DAY MEAL PLAN

Day 1:

- ✓ Breakfast: Greek Yogurt Parfait with Berries
- ✓ Lunch: Quinoa Salad with Lemon Herb Vinaigrette
- ✓ Dinner: Grilled Lemon Garlic Chicken with Roasted Vegetables
- ✓ Snack: Carrot Sticks with Hummus

Day 2:

- ✓ Breakfast: Berry Citrus Smoothie Bowl
- ✓ Lunch: Mushroom and Thyme Quinoa
- ✓ Dinner: Baked Salmon with Cauliflower Mash
- ✓ Snack: Mixed Nuts and Seeds

Day 3:

- ✓ Breakfast: Carrot-Apple-Ginger Oatmeal
- ✓ Lunch: Spinach and Feta Stuffed Chicken Breast
- ✓ Dinner: Vegetarian Zucchini Noodles with Pesto
- ✓ Snack: Sliced Cucumber with Cream Cheese

Day 4:

- ✓ Breakfast: Beetroot and Berry Chia Pudding
- ✓ Lunch: Hearty Lentil Soup
- ✓ Dinner: Grilled Turkey Burgers with Avocado Salad
- ✓ Snack: Greek Yogurt with a sprinkle of Chia Seeds

Day 5:

- ✓ Breakfast: Pineapple Mint Smoothie Bowl
- ✓ Lunch: Lemon Herb Grilled Shrimp with Quinoa
- ✓ Dinner: Baked Parmesan Zucchini Fries with Grilled Chicken
- ✓ Snack: Blueberry Basil Smoothie

Day 6:

- ✓ Breakfast: Turmeric Spice Infused Oatmeal
- ✓ Lunch: Caprese Salad with Balsamic Glaze
- ✓ Dinner: Garlic Rosemary Pork Chops with Green Bean Almondine
- ✓ Snack: Sliced Apple with Almond Butter

Day 7:

- ✓ Breakfast: Cucumber Ginger Smoothie Bowl
- ✓ Lunch: Tomato Avocado Salad with Grilled Chicken
- ✓ Dinner: Salmon and Asparagus Foil Pack
- ✓ Snack: Celery Sticks with Peanut Butter

Day 8:

- ✓ Breakfast: Lemon Herb Cauliflower Rice Bowl
- ✓ Lunch: Kale and Quinoa Stuffed Peppers
- ✓ Dinner: Turkey and Vegetable Skewers with Cauliflower Mash
- ✓ Snack: Cherry Tomatoes with Mozzarella

Day 9:

- ✓ Breakfast: Tomato Avocado Toast
- ✓ Lunch: Mediterranean Chickpea Salad
- ✓ Dinner: Baked Cod with Lemon Dill Sauce and Steamed Broccoli
- ✓ Snack: Almond and Coconut Energy Bites

Day 10:

- ✓ Breakfast: Lemon Blueberry Overnight Oats
- ✓ Lunch: Cauliflower and Chickpea Curry
- ✓ Dinner: Grilled Chicken Caesar Salad
- ✓ Snack: Sugar-Free Jello with Berries

Day 11:

- ✓ Breakfast: Peach and Almond Yogurt Bowl
- ✓ Lunch: Zucchini Noodles with Pesto and Cherry Tomatoes
- ✓ Dinner: Salmon and Spinach Stuffed Portobello Mushrooms
- ✓ Snack: Avocado Slices with Salt and Pepper

Day 12:

- ✓ Breakfast: Cinnamon Apple Chia Pudding
- ✓ Lunch: Turkey and Vegetable Stir-Fry with Cauliflower Rice
- ✓ Dinner: Eggplant and Tomato Bake with Grilled Chicken
- ✓ Snack: Cucumber Slices with Tzatziki

Day 13:

- ✓ Breakfast: Blueberry Almond Smoothie Bowl
- ✓ Lunch: Mushroom and Spinach Omelets with Sliced Strawberries
- ✓ Dinner: Vegetarian Cabbage Rolls with Tomato Sauce
- ✓ Snack: Hard-Boiled Egg with a sprinkle of Paprika

Day 14:

- ✓ Breakfast: Chia Seed and Berry Parfait
- ✓ Lunch: Chicken and Vegetable Skillet with Quinoa
- ✓ Dinner: Grilled Shrimp and Avocado Salad
- ✓ Snack: Roasted Pumpkin Seeds

Day 15:

- ✓ Breakfast: Mango Turmeric Smoothie Bowl
- ✓ Lunch: Broccoli and Cheese Stuffed Chicken Breast
- ✓ Dinner: Stir-Fried Tofu with Bok Choy and Sesame Seeds
- ✓ Snack: Celery Sticks with Creamy Peanut Butter

Day 16:

- ✓ Breakfast: Cranberry Cinnamon Spice Oatmeal
- ✓ Lunch: Spinach and Feta Turkey Burgers
- ✓ Dinner: Roasted Brussels Sprouts and Walnut Salad with Grilled Chicken
- ✓ Snack: Cheese and Cherry Tomato Skewers

Day 17:

- ✓ Breakfast: Papaya Mint Yogurt Bowl
- ✓ Lunch: Quinoa and Black Bean Stuffed Bell Peppers
- ✓ Dinner: Baked Tilapia with Lemon Dill Sauce and Asparagus
- ✓ Snack: Greek Yogurt with Cinnamon

Day 18:

- ✓ Breakfast: Kale Berry Protein Boost Smoothie Bowl
- ✓ Lunch: Caprese Stuffed Avocado
- ✓ Dinner: Vegetarian Eggplant Lasagna
- ✓ Snack: Sliced Bell Peppers with Hummus

Day 19:

- ✓ Breakfast: Apple Cinnamon Spice Delight Oatmeal
- ✓ Lunch: Lemon Garlic Shrimp and Zucchini Noodles
- ✓ Dinner: Grilled Turkey Meatballs with Cauliflower Mash
- ✓ Snack: Berries and Whipped Cream

Day 20:

- ✓ Breakfast: Melon Mint Smoothie Bowl
- ✓ Lunch: Turkey and Avocado Lettuce Wraps
- ✓ Dinner: Sautéed Spinach and Mushroom Stuffed Chicken Breast
- ✓ Snack: Cherry Tomatoes with Cottage Cheese

Day 21:

- ✓ Breakfast: Ginger Pear Energizer Smoothie Bowl
- ✓ Lunch: Mediterranean Chickpea Wrap
- ✓ Dinner: Baked Cod with Tomato and Olive Relish
- ✓ Snack: Almond Butter and Banana Slices

Day 22:

- ✓ Breakfast: Orange Carrot Glow Smoothie Bowl
- ✓ Lunch: Chicken and Vegetable Skewers with Quinoa
- ✓ Dinner: Stuffed Bell Peppers with Ground Turkey and Cauliflower Rice
- ✓ Snack: Hard-Boiled Egg with a sprinkle of Salt

Day 23:

- ✓ Breakfast: Coconut Berry Bliss Smoothie Bowl
- ✓ Lunch: Avocado and Shrimp Salad
- ✓ Dinner: Turkey and Vegetable Stir-Fry with Broccoli Rice
- ✓ Snack: Cucumber Slices with Guacamole

Day 24:

- ✓ Breakfast: Pomegranate Basil Infusion Smoothie Bowl
- ✓ Lunch: Mushroom and Spinach Frittata
- ✓ Dinner: Grilled Chicken with Tomato and Basil Salsa
- ✓ Snack: Greek Yogurt with a sprinkle of Walnuts

Day 25:

- ✓ Breakfast: Mango Turmeric Smoothie Bowl
- ✓ Lunch: Quinoa and Black Bean Salad
- ✓ Dinner: Baked Salmon with Lemon Herb Quinoa
- ✓ Snack: Mixed Berries with Cottage Cheese

Day 26:

- ✓ Breakfast: Cranberry Cinnamon Spice Oatmeal
- ✓ Lunch: Chicken and Vegetable Skillet with Cauliflower Rice
- ✓ Dinner: Grilled Shrimp and Asparagus Salad
- ✓ Snack: Sliced Apple with Almond Butter

Day 27:

- ✓ Breakfast: Blueberry Almond Smoothie Bowl
- ✓ Lunch: Caprese Stuffed Bell Peppers
- ✓ Dinner: Vegetarian Cauliflower Fried Rice with Tofu
- ✓ Snack: Carrot Sticks with Hummus

Day 28:

- ✓ Breakfast: Pineapple Mint Smoothie Bowl
- ✓ Lunch: Greek Salad with Grilled Chicken
- ✓ Dinner: Baked Cod with Mediterranean Salsa
- ✓ Snack: Mixed Nuts and Seeds

CONCLUSION

As our shared adventure through "Type 2 Diabetes Cookbook for Seniors" draws to a close, I find my heart brimming with gratitude and hope. With each turn of the page, we've woven a tapestry of flavors, stories, and, most importantly, transformations. We've embraced the dance of life, the sweet symphony of renewal, and the vibrant hues of health.

In the gentle caress of every recipe, we've discovered more than just a meal. We've uncovered the whispers of nourishment, the harmonies of balance, and the melodies of vitality. Through the tales of Martha and the kitchen symphonies, we've witnessed the magical alchemy that occurs when food becomes not just sustenance but a celebration of life.

As you bid adieu to these pages, let the echoes of these culinary journeys linger in your kitchen like the fragrance of a comforting meal. May the memories of flavors shared with loved ones become the foundation of a life well-lived and may the benefits of embracing healthy choices reverberate through your being.

In the quiet moments before a simmering pot or the gentle whisking of a vinaigrette, remember the questions stirred within your soul. What does it mean to savor life's precious moments? How does the food we choose compose the soundtrack of our existence? How can a cookbook be more than a guide—it can be a vessel of transformation?

I invite you, dear reader, to share your thoughts, your stories, and your experiences. Your feedback is not merely a collection of words but a melody that resonates within the heart of our shared journey. Let us continue to dance through the kitchen of life, refining our steps, embracing the nourishment that comes from shared stories, and encouraging one another to savor the beauty of each day.

Your insights, like the secret ingredients in a cherished family recipe, are the essence that makes our culinary tapestry richer, deeper, and more flavorful. Reach out, share your anecdotes, your discoveries, and your reflections. Together, we'll create a chorus of voices, a chorus of renewed spirits.

As you embark on your own culinary adventures beyond these pages, remember that each meal is a canvas, and you are the artist of your health. May the melodies of good health, the rhythms of joy, and the harmonies of vitality accompany you on this continued journey.

With heartfelt gratitude and anticipation for the stories yet to unfold.

BONUS CHAPTER

20 JUICING RECIPES

Green Goddess Detox Juice

Preparation Time: 10 minutes

Serving: 2

Ingredients:

- ✓ 2 cups kale, stems removed
- ✓ 1 cucumber, peeled
- ✓ 1 green apple, cored
- ✓ 1/2 lemon, peeled
- ✓ 1-inch ginger, peeled

Instructions:

1. Juice kale, cucumber, apple, lemon, and ginger.
2. Pour into glasses and enjoy this nutrient-packed, low-carb detoxifying green juice.

Nutritional Information:

80 calories, 20g carbs, 2g protein, 0.5g fat, 5g fiber.

A refreshing green juice rich in antioxidants and vitamins, promoting overall well-being and supporting a healthy metabolism.

Berry Citrus Blast

Preparation Time: 15 minutes

Serving: 2

Ingredients:

- ✓ 1 cup blueberries
- ✓ 1 cup strawberries, hulled
- ✓ 1 orange, peeled
- ✓ 1/2 lime, peeled
- ✓ 1 cup spinach

Instructions:

1. Juice blueberries, strawberries, orange, lime, and spinach.
2. Pour into glasses for a delicious, low-sugar berry and citrus explosion with a boost of vitamins.

Nutritional Information:

100 calories, 25g carbs, 2g protein, 0.5g fat, 7g fiber.

A vibrant and flavorful juice loaded with berries and citrus to satisfy sweet cravings while providing essential nutrients.

Carrot-Apple-Ginger Elixir

Preparation Time: 12 minutes

Serving: 2

Ingredients:

- ✓ 4 carrots, peeled
- ✓ 2 apples, cored
- ✓ 1-inch ginger, peeled

Instructions:

1. Juice carrots, apples, and ginger.
2. Pour into glasses for a zesty, vitamin-rich elixir that supports digestion and provides a natural energy boost.

Nutritional Information:

120 calories, 30g carbs, 1g protein, 0.5g fat, 8g fiber.

An invigorating juice combining carrots, apples, and ginger to create a flavorful elixir packed with immune-boosting properties.

Beetroot and Berry Bliss

Preparation Time: 15 minutes

Serving: 2

Ingredients:

- ✓ 1 medium beet, peeled
- ✓ 1 cup raspberries
- ✓ 1 cup blackberries
- ✓ 1/2 cup Greek yogurt (unsweetened)
- ✓ 1 tablespoon chia seeds

Instructions:

1. Juice beet, raspberries, and blackberries.
2. Blend juice with Greek yogurt and chia seeds for a delightful and fiber-rich beetroot and berry smoothie.

Nutritional Information:

140 calories, 25g carbs, 4g protein, 2g fat, 10g fiber.

A vibrant and satisfying juice blend featuring beets and berries, providing a natural sweetness and a dose of antioxidants.

Pineapple Mint Refresher

Preparation Time: 10 minutes

Serving: 2

Ingredients:

- ✓ 1 cup pineapple chunks
- ✓ 1/2 cucumber, peeled
- ✓ 1/4 cup fresh mint leaves
- ✓ 1 lime, peeled
- ✓ 1 celery stalk

Instructions:

1. Juice pineapple, cucumber, mint, lime, and celery.
2. Serve over ice for a hydrating and tropical pineapple mint refresher with a burst of citrus.

Nutritional Information:

90 calories, 22g carbs, 1g protein, 0.5g fat, 4g fiber.

A revitalizing juice with the tropical sweetness of pineapple and the refreshing essence of mint, perfect for hydration.

Turmeric Spice Infusion

Preparation Time: 12 minutes

Serving: 2

Ingredients:

- ✓ 2 large carrots, peeled
- ✓ 1 orange, peeled
- ✓ 1-inch turmeric root, peeled
- ✓ 1/2 lemon, peeled
- ✓ 1 teaspoon honey (optional)

Instructions:

1. Juice carrots, orange, turmeric, and lemon.
2. Stir in honey for a warming and anti-inflammatory turmeric spice infusion.

Nutritional Information:

110 calories, 28g carbs, 2g protein, 0.5g fat, 6g fiber.

A golden-hued juice featuring turmeric, known for its anti-inflammatory properties, offering a flavorful and healthful elixir.

Cucumber Ginger Cooler

Preparation Time: 10 minutes

Serving: 2

Ingredients:

- ✓ 2 cucumbers, peeled
- ✓ 1-inch ginger, peeled
- ✓ 1/2 lime, peeled
- ✓ 1 tablespoon fresh basil leaves
- ✓ 1 teaspoon agave syrup (optional)

Instructions:

1. Juice cucumbers, ginger, lime, and basil.
2. Sweeten with agave syrup if desired, creating a hydrating and cooling cucumber ginger cooler.

Nutritional Information:

60 calories, 15g carbs, 2g protein, 0.5g fat, 3g fiber.

A crisp and refreshing juice with cucumber and ginger, providing a cooling sensation and a touch of sweetness.

Citrus Beet Detoxifier

Preparation Time: 15 minutes

Serving: 2

Ingredients:

- ✓ 2 medium beets, peeled
- ✓ 2 oranges, peeled
- ✓ 1 grapefruit, peeled
- ✓ 1 tablespoon flaxseeds

Instructions:

1. Juice beets, oranges, and grapefruit.
2. Blend in flaxseeds for a detoxifying and fiber-packed citrus beet smoothie.

Nutritional Information:

130 calories, 30g carbs, 3g protein, 1g fat, 8g fiber.

A vibrant juice combining beets and citrus fruits, enhanced with flaxseeds for a nutritious and detoxifying beverage.

Spinach Pineapple Zinger

Preparation Time: 12 minutes

Serving: 2

Ingredients:

- ✓ 2 cups fresh spinach
- ✓ 1 cup pineapple chunks
- ✓ 1 green apple, cored
- ✓ 1/2 cucumber, peeled
- ✓ 1/2 lemon, peeled

Instructions:

1. Juice spinach, pineapple, apple, cucumber, and lemon.
2. Savor this green zinger, rich in vitamins and antioxidants, perfect for a refreshing pick-me-up.

Nutritional Information:

100 calories, 25g carbs, 2g protein, 0.5g fat, 6g fiber.

A nutrient-packed green juice combining spinach, pineapple, and apple, creating a zesty and invigorating blend.

Blueberry Basil Bliss

Preparation Time: 10 minutes

Serving: 2

Ingredients:

- ✓ 2 cups blueberries
- ✓ 1/2 cup fresh basil leaves
- ✓ 1/2 lime, peeled.
- ✓ 1 tablespoon chia seeds
- ✓ 1 teaspoon honey (optional)

Instructions:

1. Juice blueberries, basil, and lime.
2. Blend in chia seeds and sweeten with honey if desired, offering a delightful blueberry basil smoothie.

Nutritional Information:

110 calories, 25g carbs, 2g protein, 1g fat, 8g fiber.

A refreshing and antioxidant-rich blueberry basil smoothie, providing a burst of flavor and natural sweetness.

Mango Turmeric Elixir

Preparation Time: 12 minutes

Serving: 2

Ingredients:

- ✓ 1 cup mango chunks
- ✓ 1-inch turmeric root, peeled
- ✓ 1/2 orange, peeled
- ✓ 1 tablespoon flaxseeds
- ✓ 1 teaspoon honey (optional)

Instructions:

1. Juice mango, turmeric, and orange.
2. Blend in flaxseeds and sweeten with honey if desired, creating a tropical and anti-inflammatory elixir.

Nutritional Information:

140 calories, 30g carbs, 2g protein, 1g fat, 7g fiber.

A vibrant and tropical elixir featuring mango and turmeric, providing a burst of flavor and potential anti-inflammatory benefits.

Cranberry Cinnamon Spice

Preparation Time: 15 minutes

Serving: 2

Ingredients:

- ✓ 1 cup fresh cranberries
- ✓ 1 apple, cored.
- ✓ 1/2 teaspoon ground cinnamon
- ✓ 1/2 lemon, peeled.
- ✓ 1 tablespoon chia seeds

Instructions:

1. Juice cranberries, apple, cinnamon, and lemon.
2. Blend in chia seeds, creating a festive and antioxidant-rich cranberry cinnamon spice smoothie.

Nutritional Information:

120 calories, 28g carbs, 2g protein, 1g fat, 9g fiber.

A seasonal and spiced juice featuring cranberries and cinnamon, offering a flavorful and fiber-packed beverage.

Papaya Mint Cooler

Preparation Time: 10 minutes

Serving: 2

Ingredients:

- ✓ 1 cup papaya chunks
- ✓ 1/4 cup fresh mint leaves
- ✓ 1/2 lime, peeled
- ✓ 1/2 cucumber, peeled
- ✓ 1 teaspoon agave syrup (optional)

Instructions:

1. Juice papaya, mint, lime, and cucumber.
2. Sweeten with agave syrup if desired, creating a refreshing and tropical papaya mint cooler.

Nutritional Information:

100 calories, 22g carbs, 1g protein, 0.5g fat, 5g fiber.

A cooling and hydrating juice featuring papaya and mint, offering a taste of the tropics with a hint of sweetness.

Kale Berry Protein Boost

Preparation Time: 12 minutes

Serving: 2

Ingredients:

- ✓ 2 cups kale, stems removed
- ✓ 1 cup mixed berries (strawberries, blueberries, raspberries)
- ✓ 1/2 cup Greek yogurt (unsweetened)
- ✓ 1 tablespoon almond butter
- ✓ 1 teaspoon chia seeds

Instructions:

1. Juice kale and berries.
2. Blend in Greek yogurt, almond butter, and chia seeds for a protein-packed and nutrient-rich kale berry smoothie.

Nutritional Information:

160 calories, 22g carbs, 8g protein, 6g fat, 7g fiber.

A robust and satisfying smoothie featuring kale and mixed berries, providing a balance of protein and vitamins for a wholesome treat.

Apple Cinnamon Spice Delight

Preparation Time: 10 minutes

Serving: 2

Ingredients:

- ✓ 2 apples, cored
- ✓ 1/2 teaspoon ground cinnamon
- ✓ 1/4 teaspoon nutmeg
- ✓ 1/2 lemon, peeled
- ✓ 1 tablespoon flaxseeds

Instructions:

1. Juice apples, cinnamon, nutmeg, and lemon.
2. Blend in flaxseeds for a comforting and spiced apple cinnamon delight, perfect for fall-inspired refreshment.

Nutritional Information:

110 calories, 25g carbs, 1g protein, 0.5g fat, 6g fiber.

A warming and autumn-inspired juice featuring apples and cinnamon, offering a delightful blend of flavors.

Melon Mint Hydration

Preparation Time: 10 minutes

Serving: 2

Ingredients:

- ✓ 2 cups melon chunks (cantaloupe, honeydew)
- ✓ 1/4 cup fresh mint leaves
- ✓ 1/2 lime, peeled
- ✓ 1 tablespoon chia seeds

Instructions:

1. Juice melon, mint, and lime.
2. Blend in chia seeds for a hydrating and minty melon infusion, perfect for a refreshing pick-me-up.

Nutritional Information:

90 calories, 20g carbs, 2g protein, 0.5g fat, 6g fiber.

A cooling and rejuvenating juice featuring melon and mint, providing hydration with a burst of natural sweetness.

Ginger Pear Energizer

Preparation Time: 12 minutes

Serving: 2

Ingredients:

- ✓ 2 pears, cored
- ✓ 1-inch ginger, peeled
- ✓ 1/2 lemon, peeled
- ✓ 1 tablespoon hemp seeds
- ✓ 1 teaspoon honey (optional)

Instructions:

1. Juice pears, ginger, and lemon.
2. Blend in hemp seeds and sweeten with honey if desired, creating an energizing and nutrient-dense ginger pear smoothie.

Nutritional Information:

130 calories, 30g carbs, 2g protein, 1g fat, 7g fiber.

An invigorating and flavorful smoothie featuring ginger and pears, offering a natural energy boost with a touch of sweetness.

Orange Carrot Glow

Preparation Time: 10 minutes

Serving: 2

Ingredients:

- ✓ 3 oranges, peeled
- ✓ 4 carrots, peeled
- ✓ 1-inch turmeric root, peeled
- ✓ 1 tablespoon chia seeds

Instructions:

1. Juice oranges, carrots, and turmeric.
2. Blend in chia seeds for a vibrant and nutrient-packed orange carrot glow, providing a dose of vitamins and antioxidants.

Nutritional Information:

120 calories, 28g carbs, 2g protein, 0.5g fat, 9g fiber.

A refreshing and glowing juice featuring oranges, carrots, and turmeric, offering a burst of color and healthful benefits.

Coconut Berry Bliss

Preparation Time: 15 minutes

Serving: 2

Ingredients:

- ✓ 1 cup mixed berries (strawberries, blueberries, raspberries)
- ✓ 1/2 cup coconut water
- ✓ 1/2 cup Greek yogurt (unsweetened)
- ✓ 1 tablespoon chia seeds

Instructions:

1. Juice mixed berries.
2. Blend in coconut water, Greek yogurt, and chia seeds for a creamy and tropical coconut berry smoothie.

Nutritional Information:

140 calories, 20g carbs, 6g protein, 4g fat, 8g fiber.

A luscious and coconut-infused smoothie featuring mixed berries, offering a delightful combination of flavors and textures.

Pomegranate Basil Infusion

Preparation Time: 12 minutes

Serving: 2

Ingredients:

- ✓ 1 cup pomegranate seeds
- ✓ 1/4 cup fresh basil leaves
- ✓ 1/2 lime, peeled
- ✓ 1/2 cucumber, peeled
- ✓ 1 teaspoon honey (optional)

Instructions:

1. Juice pomegranate seeds, basil, lime, and cucumber.
2. Sweeten with honey if desired, creating a refreshing and antioxidant-rich pomegranate basil infusion.

Nutritional Information:

100 calories, 22g carbs, 1g protein, 0.5g fat, 5g fiber.

An antioxidant-packed and refreshing infusion featuring pomegranate and basil, offering a unique and healthful beverage.

MEAL PLANNER JOURNAL

WEEKLY PLANNER

MONDAY

TUESDAY

WEDNESDAY

THURSDAY

FRIDAY

SATUREDAY

SUNDAY

NOTE

WEEKLY PLANNER

MONDAY

TUESDAY

WEDNESDAY

THURSDAY

FRIDAY

SATUREDAY

SUNDAY

NOTE

WEEKLY PLANNER

MONDAY

TUESDAY

WEDNESDAY

THURSDAY

FRIDAY

SATUREDAY

SUNDAY

NOTE

WEEKLY PLANNER

MONDAY

TUESDAY

WEDNESDAY

THURSDAY

FRIDAY

SATUREDAY

SUNDAY

NOTE

WEEKLY PLANNER

MONDAY

TUESDAY

WEDNESDAY

THURSDAY

FRIDAY

SATUREDAY

SUNDAY

NOTE

WEEKLY PLANNER

MONDAY	TUESDAY

WEDNESDAY	THURSDAY

FRIDAY	SATUREDAY

SUNDAY	NOTE

WEEKLY PLANNER

MONDAY

TUESDAY

WEDNESDAY

THURSDAY

FRIDAY

SATUREDAY

SUNDAY

NOTE

WEEKLY PLANNER

MONDAY	TUESDAY

WEDNESDAY	THURSDAY

FRIDAY	SATUREDAY

SUNDAY	NOTE

WEEKLY PLANNER

MONDAY

TUESDAY

WEDNESDAY

THURSDAY

FRIDAY

SATUREDAY

SUNDAY

NOTE

WEEKLY PLANNER

MONDAY	TUESDAY

WEDNESDAY	THURSDAY

FRIDAY	SATUREDAY

SUNDAY	NOTE

www.ingramcontent.com/pod-product-compliance
Lightning Source LLC
Chambersburg PA
CBHW080928260726
48661CB00010B/3845